MW01243888

Legs Plus

Workouts

By Karen Goeller, CSCS

Photos by Bossio Photography, NJ

Legs Plus Workouts

To contact the author visit…
www.KarenGoeller.com.
To contact the photographer visit…
www.BossioPhotography.com

ISBN-13: 978-1492150831

ISBN-10: 1492150835

Legs Plus Workouts

These LEGS PLUS workouts are challenging. Please discuss this new exercise program with your medical provider. If you have not exercised regularly in recent months you should start with one set of 10 repetitions each exercise. It does not sound like much, but remember, each exercise is actually two exercises combined. Once you can easily perform one set of 10 repetitions each exercise you may start to add a second round of one set of each exercise. After you are able to perform two rounds of each exercise you should also be able to perform the workouts by doing two sets of each exercise before moving on to the next exercise. The reason for doing the two rounds method before the two sets of each exercise method is to make sure you get a well-rounded workout. Another method is that you may also try performing each exercise for 15-30 seconds at a steady pace rather than for a set number of repetitions. Perform one, two, or three rounds, depending upon your fitness level.

Make sure your knees remain in line with your hip and toes. Do not allow your knee to move laterally, from side to side on any exercise. Make sure your knee does not go forward beyond your toes.

You are responsible for your personal safety. By participating in this workout you are stating that you are healthy enough to take on a strenuous fitness program. You are also stating that you have your doctor's permission to participate in a strenuous fitness program with or without a fitness trainer. **You must stop if you feel pain, dizzy, nauseous, injured, or ill.**

WARNING: Any activity involving motion creates the possibility of accidental injury, paralysis or death. These instructional materials are intended for use ONLY by properly trained and qualified participants under supervised conditions. Use without proper supervision or knowledge could be DANGEROUS and should NOT be undertaken or permitted. Before using, KNOW YOUR OWN LIMITATIONS and the limitations of your equipment. If in doubt always consult an instructor. Always inspect equipment for loose fittings or damage and test for stability before each use. We will not be liable for injuries or consequences sustained in the use of the instructional materials, workouts, or equipment sold by us.

Contents

Legs Plus Workouts

Legs Plus Workouts

Legs Plus Workouts

LEGS PLUS WORKOUT ONE

Legs Plus Workouts

Squat with Iron Cross

1. Use dumbbells appropriate for your fitness level. Choose the amount of weight based on your upper body strength.
2. Start standing with your feet shoulder width apart and your chest up.
3. Hold weights securely at shoulder height with palms facing forward.
4. Bend at your hips and knees as you squat
5. Push your hips back to bring your thighs to nearly parallel to the ground. Make sure your knees remain in line with your hips and toes. Do not allow your knees to move laterally, from side to side. Make sure your knees do not go forward beyond your toes.
6. As you begin to squat, bring your hands towards each other in front of your chest.
7. Hold briefly in this position and then stand up while simultaneously moving your arms out to the sides and still at shoulder height.
8. Make sure your knees remain in line with your hip and toes. Do not allow the knee to move laterally, from side to side on any exercise. Make sure your knee does not go forward beyond your toes.

Legs Plus Workouts

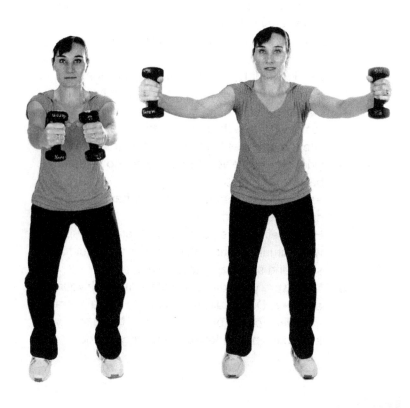

Reverse Lunge with Front Raise

1. Use dumbbells appropriate for your fitness level. Choose the amount of weight based on your upper body strength.
2. Start standing with your feet together and your chest up.
3. Hold weights securely at your thighs with palms facing body.
4. Lift left foot from floor and reach back with that foot. The goal is to bring the knee on your left leg close to floor behind you without actually touching the floor. Your left foot will touch the floor.
5. Bend the right leg as your left knee gets close to the floor.
6. As the leg is going back, bring left arm forward and up to the height of your shoulder. Bring your right arm up to the side and the height of your shoulder. Arms will be in an L position.
7. Keep your elbows relaxed, not locked.
8. Bottom position will be a lunge, both legs bent at near 90 degrees with back knee close to floor. Your arms will be in an L position at shoulder height.
9. Hold briefly in this position.
10. Return to starting position by standing back up to bring your legs together and your hands back down to your thighs.
11. Repeat this exercise with the right leg stepping back and the opposite arms.

Legs Plus Workouts

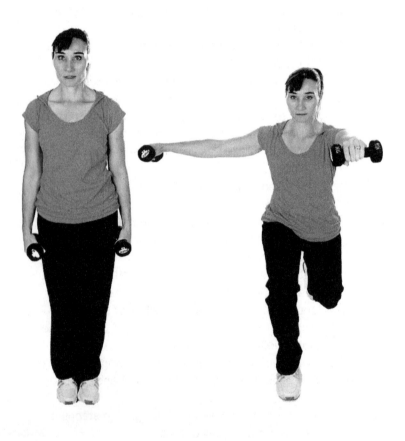

Chops

1. Use medicine ball appropriate for your fitness level. Choose the amount of weight based on your upper body strength.
2. Start standing with your feet shoulder width apart and your chest up.
3. Hold medicine ball securely in front of body.
4. Holding ball in front of body, perform a squat. Bend at your hips and knees as you squat
5. Push your hips back to bring your thighs to nearly parallel to the ground. Make sure your knees remain in line with your hips and toes. Do not allow your knees to move laterally, from side to side. Make sure your knees do not go forward beyond your toes.
6. As you rise from the squat bring the medicine ball forward and then up above your head.
7. Hold briefly in this position and then squat again while simultaneously moving your arms with the ball to the lower position in front of your body.

Legs Plus Workouts

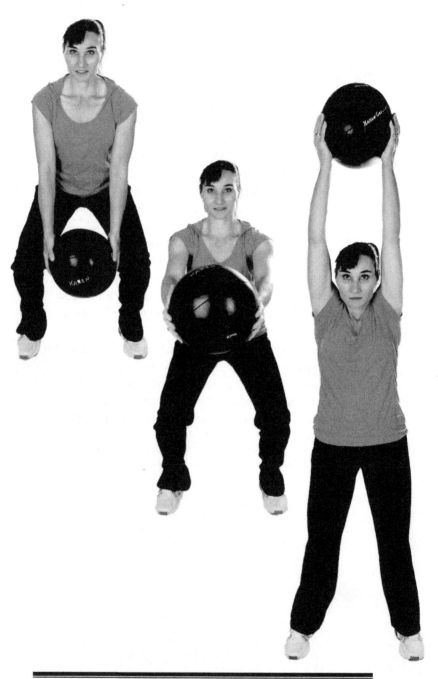

Lunge and Press

1. Use medicine ball appropriate for your fitness level. Choose the amount of weight based on your upper body strength.
2. Start standing with your feet together and your chest up. Take a step forward with your right foot, as far as comfortable without losing balance.
3. Hold medicine ball securely in front of your chest.
4. Keeping your chest up, bend both knees so that your back knee drops close to the floor.
5. The goal is to bring the knee on your left leg close to floor behind you without actually touching the floor. Your left foot will remain on the floor.
6. The thigh on your right leg will be nearly parallel to the floor at the bottom of the exercise.
7. Bottom position will be a lunge, both legs bent at near 90 degrees with back knee close to floor. The medicine ball will be in front of your chest.
8. Hold briefly in this position.
9. Begin to rise back up and simultaneously lift the ball above your head.
10. Stay tall, but do not lean back.
11. Repeat this exercise with the other leg in front.

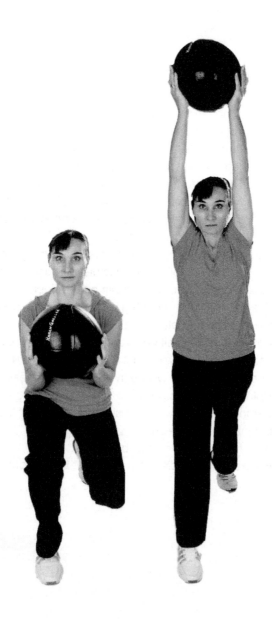

Squat with Alternating Overhead Press

1. Use dumbbells appropriate for your fitness level. Choose the amount of weight based on your upper body strength.
2. Start standing with your feet shoulder width apart and your chest up.
3. Hold dumbbells securely in front of shoulders to start.
4. Bend at your hips and knees as you squat
5. Push your hips back to bring your thighs to nearly parallel to the ground. Make sure your knees remain in line with your hips and toes. Do not allow your knees to move laterally, from side to side. Make sure your knees do not go forward beyond your toes.
6. As you rise from the squat press one dumbbell up above your head. Keep the other dumbbell in pace at your shoulder
7. Hold briefly in this position and then squat again while simultaneously moving your arm with the dumbbell to the lower position in front of your shoulder.
8. Repeat the rise and press the other dumbbell up towards the ceiling.

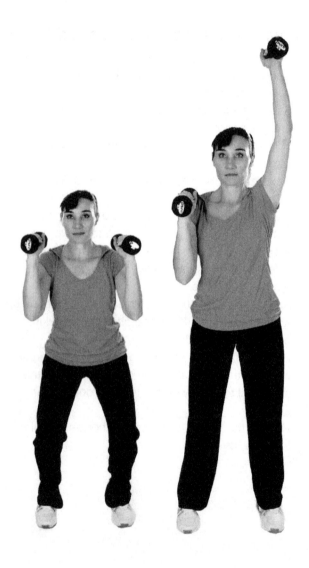

LEGS PLUS WORKOUT TWO

Legs Plus Workouts

Reverse Lunge with Front / Side Raise

1. Use dumbbells appropriate for your fitness level. Choose the amount of weight based on your upper body strength.
2. Start standing with your feet together and your chest up.
3. Hold weights securely at your thighs with palms facing body.
4. Lift left foot from floor and reach back with that foot. The goal is to bring the knee on your left leg close to floor behind you without actually touching the floor. Your left foot will touch the floor.
5. Bend the right leg as your left knee gets close to the floor.
6. As the leg is going back, bring left arm forward and up to the height of your shoulder. Bring your right arm up to the side and the height of your shoulder. Arms will be in an L position.
7. Keep your elbows relaxed, not locked.
8. Bottom position will be a lunge, both legs bent at near 90 degrees with back knee close to floor. Your arms will be in an L position at shoulder height.
9. Hold briefly in this position.
10. Return to starting position by standing back up to bring your legs together and your hands back down to your thighs.
11. Repeat this exercise with the right leg stepping back and the opposite arms.

Legs Plus Workouts

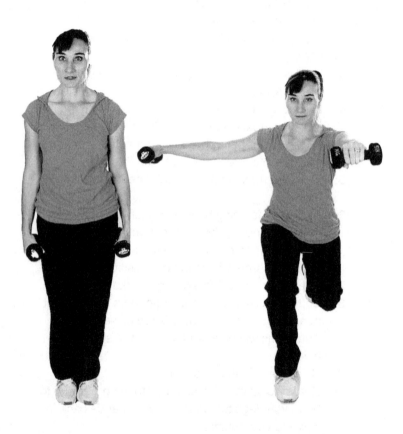

Squat with Row

1. Use dumbbells appropriate for your fitness level. Choose the amount of weight based on your upper body strength.
2. Start standing with your feet shoulder width apart and your chest up.
3. Hold dumbbells securely in at your sides to start.
4. Bend at your hips and knees as you squat
5. Push your hips back to bring your thighs to nearly parallel to the ground. Make sure your knees remain in line with your hips and toes. Do not allow your knees to move laterally, from side to side. Make sure your knees do not go forward beyond your toes.
6. As you rise from the squat pull the dumbbells up towards your hips in a rowing motion.
7. Hold briefly in this position and then squat again while simultaneously moving your arms with the dumbbells to the lower position.
8. Repeat the rise and press the other dumbbell up towards the ceiling.

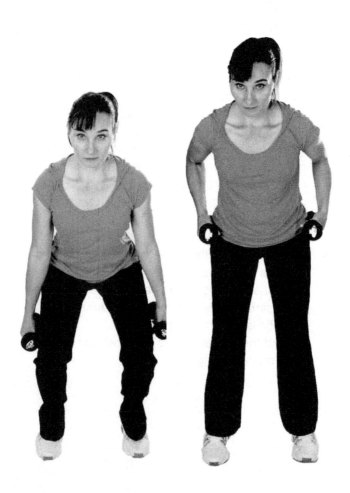

Lunge with Crossover

1. Use medicine ball appropriate for your fitness level. Choose the amount of weight based on your upper body strength.
2. Start standing with your feet together and your chest up. Take a step forward with your right foot, as far as comfortable without losing balance.
3. Hold medicine ball securely in front of your body, to start. Once you bend your legs, the medicine ball should be inside your front thigh.
4. Keeping your chest up, bend both knees so that your back knee drops close to the floor.
5. The goal is to bring the knee on your left leg close to floor behind you without actually touching the floor. Your left foot will remain on the floor.
6. The thigh on your right leg will be nearly parallel to the floor at the bottom of the exercise.
7. Bottom position will be a lunge, both legs bent at near 90 degrees with back knee close to floor. The medicine ball will be in front of your body, inside your front thigh.
8. Hold briefly in this position.
9. Begin to rise up and simultaneously lift the ball forward and then above your opposite shoulder.
10. Stay tall, but do not lean back.
11. Repeat this exercise with the other leg in front.

Legs Plus Workouts

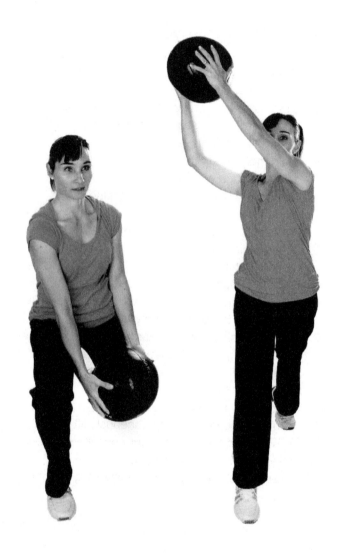

Squat and Press with Medicine Ball

1. Use medicine ball appropriate for your fitness level. Choose the amount of weight based on your upper body strength.
2. Start standing with your feet shoulder width apart and your chest up.
3. Hold medicine ball securely in front of chest.
4. Perform a squat. Bend at your hips and knees as you squat Simultaneously lower the medicine ball so that it is between your legs at a comfortable position.
5. Push your hips back to bring your thighs to nearly parallel to the ground. Make sure your knees remain in line with your hips and toes. Do not allow your knees to move laterally, from side to side. Make sure your knees do not go forward beyond your toes.
6. As you rise from the squat bring the medicine ball forward , in front of your chest, and then up above your head.
7. Hold briefly in this position and then squat again while simultaneously moving your arms with the ball to your chest and then the lower position in front of your body.

Legs Plus Workouts

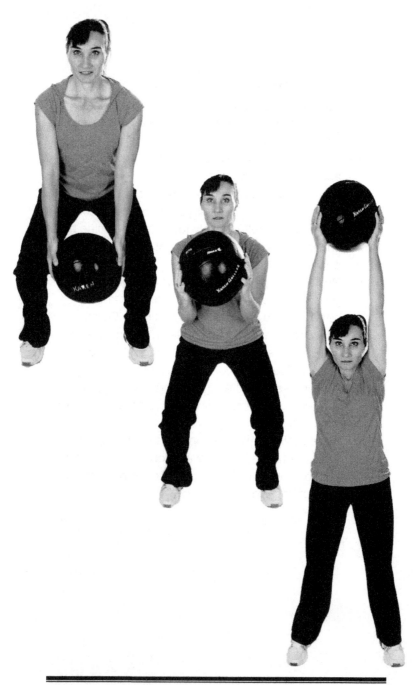

Lunge and Curl

1. Use dumbbells appropriate for your fitness level. Choose the amount of weight based on your upper body strength.
2. Start standing with your feet together and your chest up. Take a step forward with your right foot, as far as comfortable without losing balance.
3. Hold dumbbells securely at your sides.
4. Keeping your chest up, bend both knees so that your back knee drops close to the floor.
5. The goal is to bring the knee on your left leg close to floor behind you without actually touching the floor. Your left foot will remain on the floor.
6. The thigh on your right leg will be nearly parallel to the floor at the bottom of the exercise.
7. Bottom position will be a lunge, both legs bent at near 90 degrees with back knee close to floor. The dumbbells will be at your sides.
8. Hold briefly in this position.
9. Begin to rise back up and simultaneously curl the dumbbells so that your arms bend to a 90 degree angle. Keep your elbows pressed on your body so that you are performing a controlled biceps curl.
10. Stay tall, but do not lean back.
11. Repeat this exercise with the other leg in front.

Legs Plus Workouts

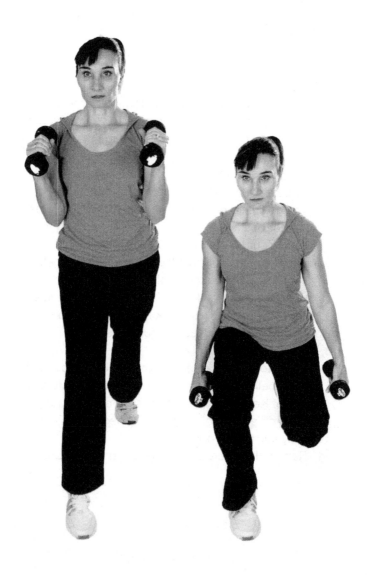

LEGS PLUS WORKOUT THREE

Legs Plus Workouts

Legs Plus Workouts

Chops

1. Use medicine ball appropriate for your fitness level. Choose the amount of weight based on your upper body strength.
2. Start standing with your feet shoulder width apart and your chest up.
3. Hold medicine ball securely in front of body.
4. Holding ball in front of body, perform a squat. Bend at your hips and knees as you squat
5. Push your hips back to bring your thighs to nearly parallel to the ground. Make sure your knees remain in line with your hips and toes. Do not allow your knees to move laterally, from side to side. Make sure your knees do not go forward beyond your toes.
6. As you rise from the squat bring the medicine ball forward and then up above your head.
7. Hold briefly in this position and then squat again while simultaneously moving your arms with the ball to the lower position in front of your body.

Legs Plus Workouts

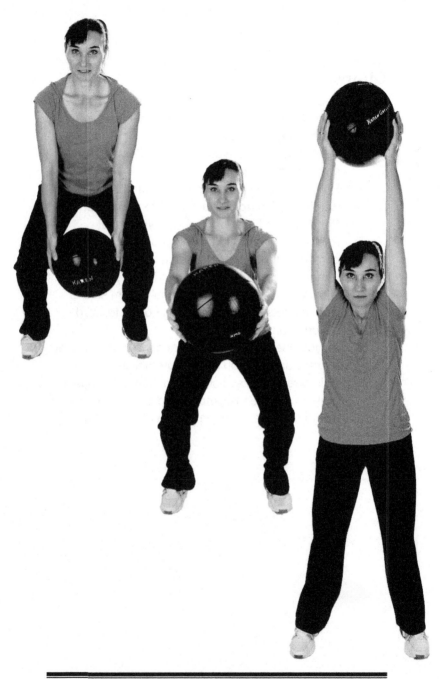

Mountain Climbers

1. Start in a push up position.
2. Your hands may be on the floor or on dumbbells that will not roll out.
3. Your body will be straight or slightly rounded, as long as your core does not fall towards the floor.
4. Bring your right knee in towards your chest, keeping your foot off the floor.
5. Switch your legs, returning the right leg to the starting position and then bringing the left knee in towards your chest.
6. You can think of this exercise as alternating knee ins or as a running motion if you are comfortable moving quickly.

Legs Plus Workouts

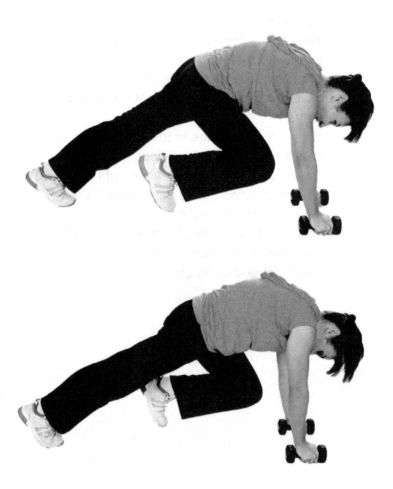

Circles

1. Use medicine ball appropriate for your fitness level. Choose the amount of weight based on your upper body strength.
2. Start standing with your feet shoulder width apart and your chest up.
3. Hold medicine ball securely in front of body.
4. Holding ball in front of body, perform a squat. Bend at your hips and knees as you squat
5. Push your hips back to bring your thighs to nearly parallel to the ground. Make sure your knees remain in line with your hips and toes. Do not allow your knees to move laterally, from side to side. Make sure your knees do not go forward beyond your toes.
6. As you rise from the squat bring the medicine ball to the right side and then up above your head.
7. Lower the medicine ball to the left side as you squat again.
8. Continue with a circular motion as you squat and rise.
9. Perform circles to the left for the same number of repetitions as you did to the right.

Legs Plus Workouts

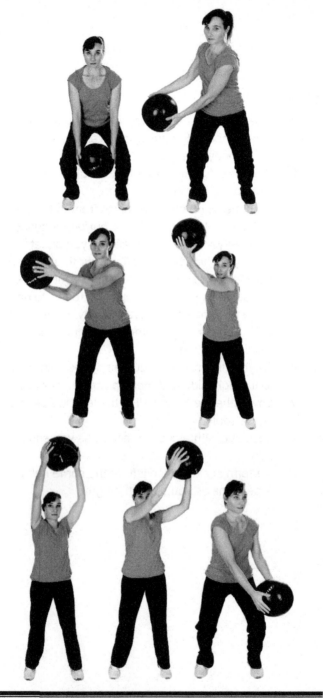

Step Up with Knee Lift

1. Stand in front of step no higher than the height of your knee.
2. Place your right foot on the step to start.
3. Bend both arms to a 90 degree angle.
4. Lift the left arm forward and up so that you will be using the opposite arm to leg motion.
5. Step up onto the step and lift your left knee towards the ceiling, keeping the left leg bent.
6. S you step up you will switch arms as if performing a marching or running motion.
7. At the top of the exercise you will be on the step with your left leg up and right arm in front.
8. Bring the left foot back towards the floor and bend that knee as your foot makes contact with the floor.
9. Repeat the exercise with the left foot on the step for the same number of repetitions as you did on the right.

Legs Plus Workouts

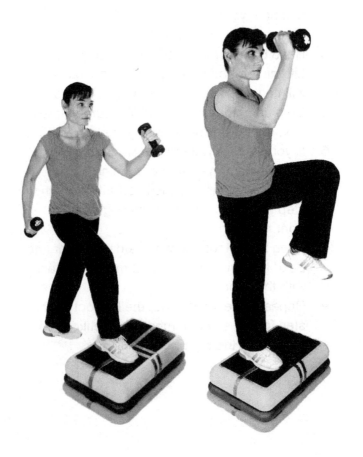

Legs Plus Workouts

Lunge with Press with Dumbbells

1. Use dumbbells appropriate for your fitness level. Choose the amount of weight based on your upper body strength.
2. Start standing with your feet together and your chest up. Take a step forward with your right foot, as far as comfortable without losing balance.
3. Hold dumbbells securely at your shoulders.
4. Keeping your chest up, bend both knees so that your back knee drops close to the floor.
5. The goal is to bring the knee on your left leg close to floor behind you without actually touching the floor. Your left foot will remain on the floor.
6. The thigh on your right leg will be nearly parallel to the floor at the bottom of the exercise.
7. Bottom position will be a lunge, both legs bent at near 90 degrees with back knee close to floor. The dumbbells will be at your shoulders.
8. Hold briefly in this position.
9. Begin to rise back up and simultaneously press the dumbbells up towards the ceiling so that the dumbbells are high above your head. Do not lock your elbows at the top.
10. Stay tall, but do not lean back.
11. Repeat this exercise with the other leg in front.

Legs Plus Workouts

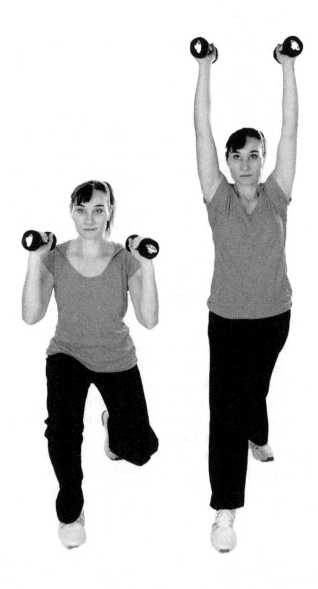

Driving

1. Use medicine ball appropriate for your fitness level. Choose the amount of weight based on your upper body strength.
2. Start standing with your feet shoulder width apart and your chest up.
3. Hold medicine ball securely in front of body at chest height.
4. Holding ball in front of body, perform a squat. Bend at your hips and knees as you squat
5. Push your hips back to bring your thighs to nearly parallel to the ground. Make sure your knees remain in line with your hips and toes. Do not allow your knees to move laterally, from side to side. Make sure your knees do not go forward beyond your toes.
6. Hold the squat position with the ball at chest height during this exercise.
7. Rotate the ball so that your right hand is on top and your left hand is on the bottom.
8. Rotate the ball again so that your left hand is on top and right hand is on bottom. Continue to rotate the ball in a driving motion as you keep it at chest height in front of your body.

Legs Plus Workouts

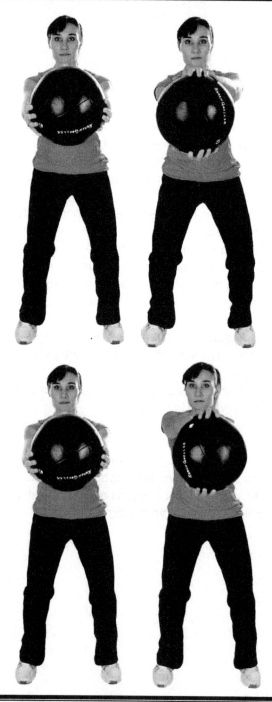

LEGS PLUS WORKOUT FOUR

Legs Plus Workouts

Squat and Upright Row

1. Use dumbbell appropriate for your fitness level. Choose the amount of weight based on your upper body strength.
2. Start standing with your feet shoulder width apart and your chest up.
3. Hold dumbbell securely in front of your body to start. Hold the inner portion of the end, rounded part of the dumbbell.
4. Bend at your hips and knees as you squat
5. Push your hips back to bring your thighs to nearly parallel to the ground. Make sure your knees remain in line with your hips and toes. Do not allow your knees to move laterally, from side to side. Make sure your knees do not go forward beyond your toes.
6. As you rise from the squat pull the dumbbell up towards your ribs. Pull to a comfortable height, no higher than chest.
7. Hold briefly in this position and then squat again while simultaneously moving your arms with the dumbbell to the lower position.

Legs Plus Workouts

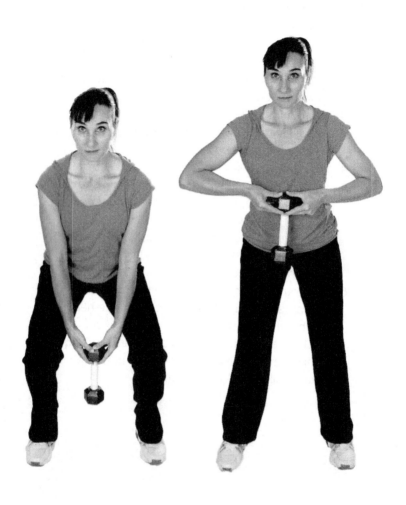

Side Lunge with Front / Side Raise

1. Use dumbbells appropriate for your fitness level. Choose the amount of weight based on your upper body strength.
2. Start standing with your feet together and your chest up.
3. Hold weights securely at your thighs with palms facing body.
4. Take a large step with right foot out to the right side.
5. As right foot makes contact with the floor, bend the knee and at the hip to form a side lunge position.
6. As the leg is stepping to the side, bring left arm forward and up to the height of your shoulder. Bring your right arm up to the side and the height of your shoulder. Arms will be in an L position.
7. Keep your elbows relaxed, not locked.
8. Bottom position will be a side lunge, right leg bent at near 90 degrees with left leg straight. Your arms will be in an L position at shoulder height.
9. Hold briefly in this position.
10. Return to starting position by standing back up to bring your legs together and your hands back down to your thighs.
11. Repeat this exercise with the left leg stepping to the left side with the opposite arms rising to shoulder height.

Legs Plus Workouts

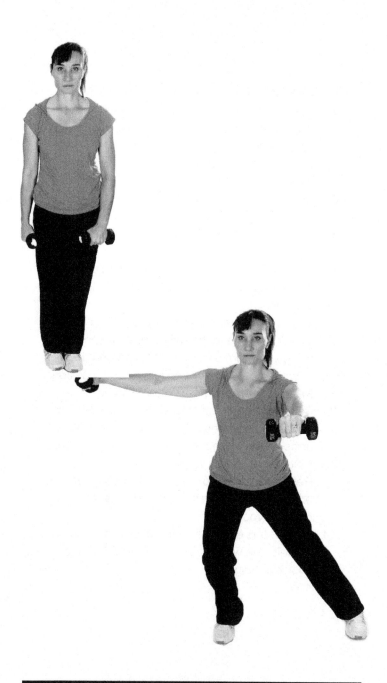

Squat and Press Medicine Ball

1. Use medicine ball appropriate for your fitness level. Choose the amount of weight based on your upper body strength.
2. Start standing with your feet shoulder width apart and your chest up.
3. Hold medicine ball securely in front of chest.
4. Perform a squat. Bend at your hips and knees as you squat Simultaneously lower the medicine ball so that it is between your legs at a comfortable position.
5. Push your hips back to bring your thighs to nearly parallel to the ground. Make sure your knees remain in line with your hips and toes. Do not allow your knees to move laterally, from side to side. Make sure your knees do not go forward beyond your toes.
6. As you rise from the squat bring the medicine ball forward , in front of your chest, and then up above your head.
7. Hold briefly in this position and then squat again while simultaneously moving your arms with the ball to your chest and then the lower position in front of your body.

Legs Plus Workouts

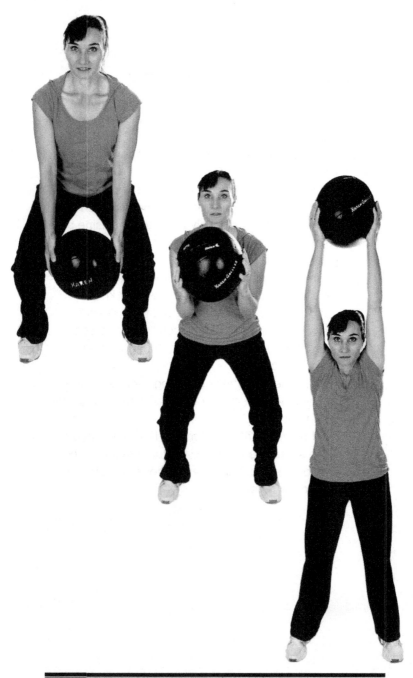

Legs Plus Workouts

Figure 8

1. Use medicine ball appropriate for your fitness level. Choose the amount of weight based on your upper body strength.
2. Start standing with your feet shoulder width apart and your chest up.
3. Hold medicine ball securely in front of body.
4. Holding ball in front of body, perform a squat. Bend at your hips and knees as you squat
5. Push your hips back to bring your thighs to nearly parallel to the ground. Make sure your knees remain in line with your hips and toes. Do not allow your knees to move laterally, from side to side. Make sure your knees do not go forward beyond your toes.
6. As you rise from the squat bring the medicine ball to the right side and then up above your head.
7. Lower the medicine ball forward so that it is in front of your chest and immediately bring it to the left thigh.
8. Squat each time the ball is lowered. Rise each time the ball is lifted.
9. Once the ball touches the thigh lift it up towards the left, above your head, forward , and to the right thigh.
10. Continue the figure 8 pattern. It will feel like you are forming two circles side by side.

Legs Plus Workouts

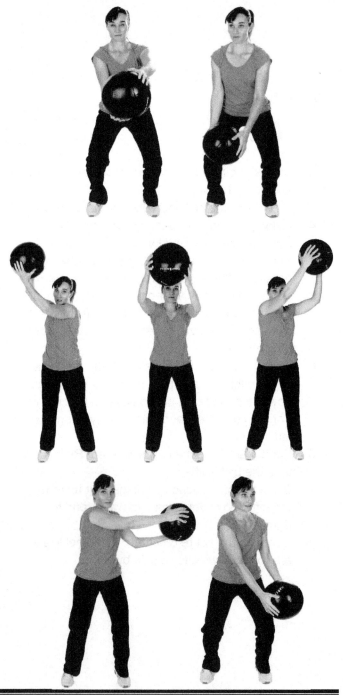

Legs Plus Workouts

Lunge and Curl

1. Use dumbbells appropriate for your fitness level. Choose the amount of weight based on your upper body strength.
2. Start standing with your feet together and your chest up. Take a step forward with your right foot, as far as comfortable without losing balance.
3. Hold dumbbells securely at your sides.
4. Keeping your chest up, bend both knees so that your back knee drops close to the floor.
5. The goal is to bring the knee on your left leg close to floor behind you without actually touching the floor. Your left foot will remain on the floor.
6. The thigh on your right leg will be nearly parallel to the floor at the bottom of the exercise.
7. Bottom position will be a lunge, both legs bent at near 90 degrees with back knee close to floor. The dumbbells will be at your sides.
8. Hold briefly in this position.
9. Begin to rise back up and simultaneously curl the dumbbells so that your arms bend to a 90 degree angle. Keep your elbows pressed on your body so that you are performing a controlled biceps curl.
10. Stay tall, but do not lean back.
11. Repeat this exercise with the other leg in front.

Legs Plus Workouts

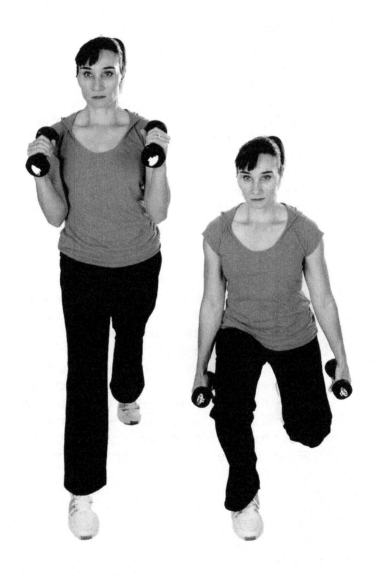

Squat and Alternating Overhead Press

1. Use dumbbells appropriate for your fitness level. Choose the amount of weight based on your upper body strength.
2. Start standing with your feet shoulder width apart and your chest up.
3. Hold dumbbells securely in front of shoulders to start.
4. Bend at your hips and knees as you squat
5. Push your hips back to bring your thighs to nearly parallel to the ground. Make sure your knees remain in line with your hips and toes. Do not allow your knees to move laterally, from side to side. Make sure your knees do not go forward beyond your toes.
6. As you rise from the squat press one dumbbell up above your head. Keep the other dumbbell in pace at your shoulder
7. Hold briefly in this position and then squat again while simultaneously moving your arm with the dumbbell to the lower position in front of your shoulder.
8. Repeat the rise and press the other dumbbell up towards the ceiling.

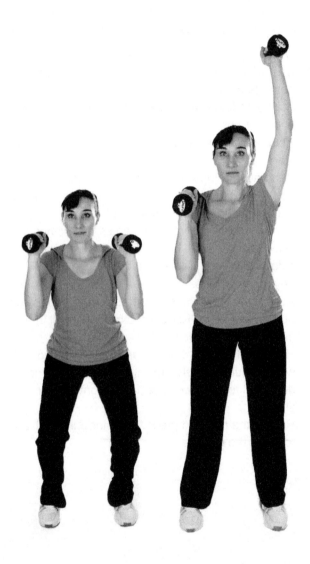

LEGS PLUS WORKOUT FIVE

Legs Plus Workouts

Squat with Iron Cross

1. Use dumbbells appropriate for your fitness level. Choose the amount of weight based on your upper body strength.
2. Start standing with your feet shoulder width apart and your chest up.
3. Hold weights securely at shoulder height with palms facing forward.
4. Bend at your hips and knees as you squat
5. Push your hips back to bring your thighs to nearly parallel to the ground. Make sure your knees remain in line with your hips and toes. Do not allow your knees to move laterally, from side to side. Make sure your knees do not go forward beyond your toes.
6. As you begin to squat, bring your hands towards each other in front of your chest.
7. Hold briefly in this position and then stand up while simultaneously moving your arms out to the sides and still at shoulder height.

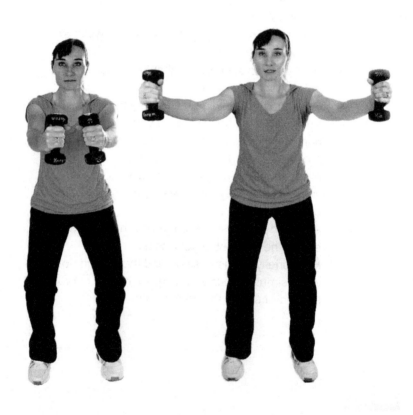

Lunge and Curl

1. Use dumbbells appropriate for your fitness level. Choose the amount of weight based on your upper body strength.
2. Start standing with your feet together and your chest up. Take a step forward with your right foot, as far as comfortable without losing balance.
3. Hold dumbbells securely at your sides.
4. Keeping your chest up, bend both knees so that your back knee drops close to the floor.
5. The goal is to bring the knee on your left leg close to floor behind you without actually touching the floor. Your left foot will remain on the floor.
6. The thigh on your right leg will be nearly parallel to the floor at the bottom of the exercise.
7. Bottom position will be a lunge, both legs bent at near 90 degrees with back knee close to floor. The dumbbells will be at your sides.
8. Hold briefly in this position.
9. Begin to rise back up and simultaneously curl the dumbbells so that your arms bend to a 90 degree angle. Keep your elbows pressed on your body so that you are performing a controlled biceps curl.
10. Stay tall, but do not lean back.
11. Repeat this exercise with the other leg in front.

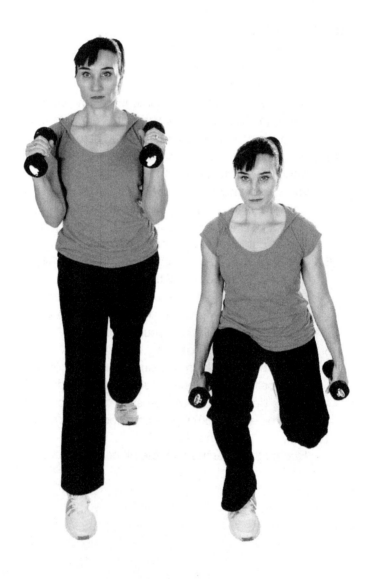

Step Up and Knee Lift

1. Stand in front of step no higher than the height of your knee.
2. Place your right foot on the step to start.
3. Bend both arms to a 90 degree angle.
4. Lift the left arm forward and up so that you will be using the opposite arm to leg motion.
5. Step up onto the step and lift your left knee towards the ceiling, keeping the left leg bent.
6. S you step up you will switch arms as if performing a marching or running motion.
7. At the top of the exercise you will be on the step with your left leg up and right arm in front.
8. Bring the left foot back towards the floor and bend that knee as your foot makes contact with the floor.
9. Repeat the exercise with the left foot on the step for the same number of repetitions as you did on the right.

Legs Plus Workouts

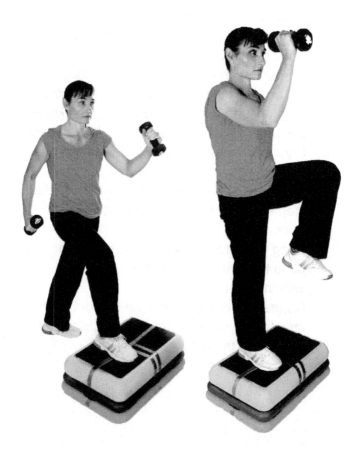

Legs Plus Workouts

Driving

1. Use medicine ball appropriate for your fitness level. Choose the amount of weight based on your upper body strength.
2. Start standing with your feet shoulder width apart and your chest up.
3. Hold medicine ball securely in front of body at chest height.
4. Holding ball in front of body, perform a squat. Bend at your hips and knees as you squat
5. Push your hips back to bring your thighs to nearly parallel to the ground. Make sure your knees remain in line with your hips and toes. Do not allow your knees to move laterally, from side to side. Make sure your knees do not go forward beyond your toes.
6. Hold the squat position with the ball at chest height during this exercise.
7. Rotate the ball so that your right hand is on top and your left hand is on the bottom.
8. Rotate the ball again so that your left hand is on top and right hand is on bottom. Continue to rotate the ball in a driving motion as you keep it at chest height in front of your body.

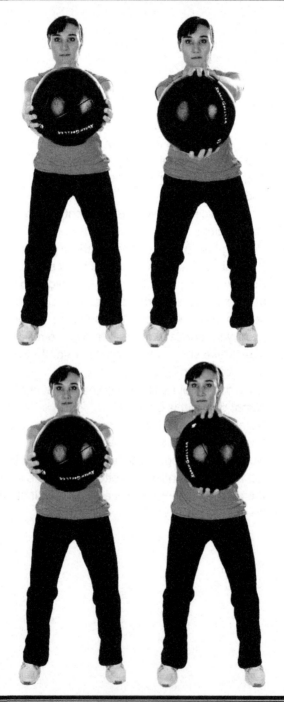

Squat and Press with Dumbbells

1. Use dumbbells appropriate for your fitness level. Choose the amount of weight based on your upper body strength.
2. Start standing with your feet shoulder width apart and your chest up.
3. Hold dumbbells securely in front of shoulders to start.
4. Bend at your hips and knees as you squat
5. Push your hips back to bring your thighs to nearly parallel to the ground. Make sure your knees remain in line with your hips and toes. Do not allow your knees to move laterally, from side to side. Make sure your knees do not go forward beyond your toes.
6. As you rise from the squat press the dumbbells up above your head.
7. Hold briefly in this position and then squat again while simultaneously moving your arms with the dumbbells to the lower position in front of your shoulders.
8. Repeat the rise and press the dumbbells up towards the ceiling.

Legs Plus Workouts

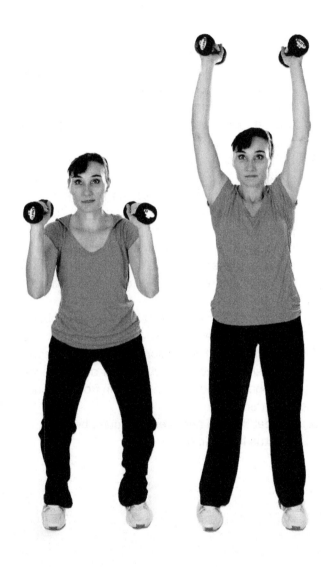

Legs Plus Workouts

Circles

1. Use medicine ball appropriate for your fitness level. Choose the amount of weight based on your upper body strength.
2. Start standing with your feet shoulder width apart and your chest up.
3. Hold medicine ball securely in front of body.
4. Holding ball in front of body, perform a squat. Bend at your hips and knees as you squat
5. Push your hips back to bring your thighs to nearly parallel to the ground. Make sure your knees remain in line with your hips and toes. Do not allow your knees to move laterally, from side to side. Make sure your knees do not go forward beyond your toes.
6. As you rise from the squat bring the medicine ball to the right side and then up above your head.
7. Lower the medicine ball to the left side as you squat again.
8. Continue with a circular motion as you squat and rise.
9. Perform circles to the left for the same number of repetitions as you did to the right.

Legs Plus Workouts

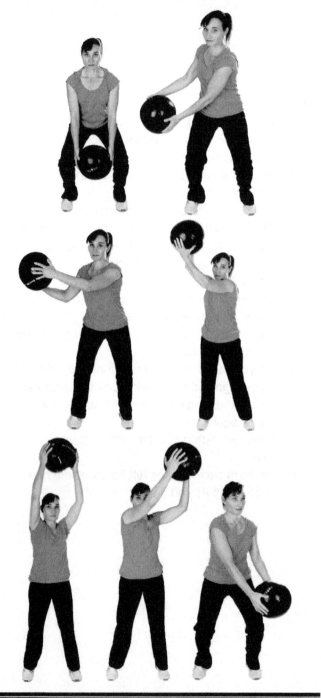

LEGS PLUS WORKOUT SIX

Legs Plus Workouts

Squat and Upright Row

1. Use dumbbell appropriate for your fitness level. Choose the amount of weight based on your upper body strength.
2. Start standing with your feet shoulder width apart and your chest up.
3. Hold dumbbell securely in front of your body to start. Hold the inner portion of the end, rounded part of the dumbbell.
4. Bend at your hips and knees as you squat
5. Push your hips back to bring your thighs to nearly parallel to the ground. Make sure your knees remain in line with your hips and toes. Do not allow your knees to move laterally, from side to side. Make sure your knees do not go forward beyond your toes.
6. As you rise from the squat pull the dumbbell up towards your ribs. Pull to a comfortable height, no higher than chest.
7. Hold briefly in this position and then squat again while simultaneously moving your arms with the dumbbell to the lower position.

Legs Plus Workouts

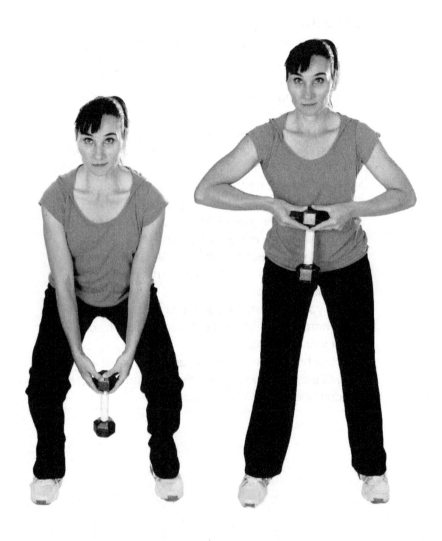

Legs Plus Workouts

Lunge and Curl

1. Use dumbbells appropriate for your fitness level. Choose the amount of weight based on your upper body strength.
2. Start standing with your feet together and your chest up. Take a step forward with your right foot, as far as comfortable without losing balance.
3. Hold dumbbells securely at your sides.
4. Keeping your chest up, bend both knees so that your back knee drops close to the floor.
5. The goal is to bring the knee on your left leg close to floor behind you without actually touching the floor. Your left foot will remain on the floor.
6. The thigh on your right leg will be nearly parallel to the floor at the bottom of the exercise.
7. Bottom position will be a lunge, both legs bent at near 90 degrees with back knee close to floor. The dumbbells will be at your sides.
8. Hold briefly in this position.
9. Begin to rise back up and simultaneously curl the dumbbells so that your arms bend to a 90 degree angle. Keep your elbows pressed on your body so that you are performing a controlled biceps curl.
10. Stay tall, but do not lean back.
11. Repeat this exercise with the other leg in front.

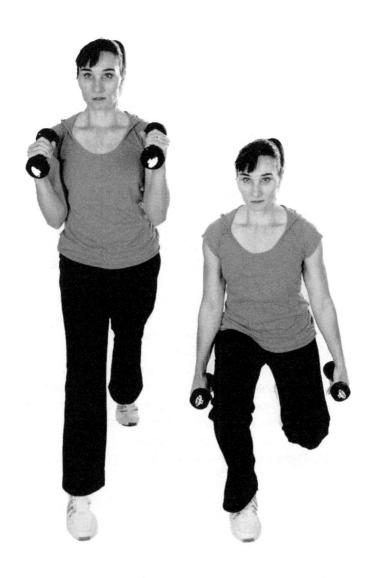

Lunge and Press

12. Use medicine ball appropriate for your fitness level. Choose the amount of weight based on your upper body strength.
13. Start standing with your feet together and your chest up. Take a step forward with your right foot, as far as comfortable without losing balance.
14. Hold medicine ball securely in front of your chest.
15. Keeping your chest up, bend both knees so that your back knee drops close to the floor.
16. The goal is to bring the knee on your left leg close to floor behind you without actually touching the floor. Your left foot will remain on the floor.
17. The thigh on your right leg will be nearly parallel to the floor at the bottom of the exercise.
18. Bottom position will be a lunge, both legs bent at near 90 degrees with back knee close to floor. The medicine ball will be in front of your chest.
19. Hold briefly in this position.
20. Begin to rise back up and simultaneously lift the ball above your head.
21. Stay tall, but do not lean back.
22. Repeat this exercise with the other leg in front.

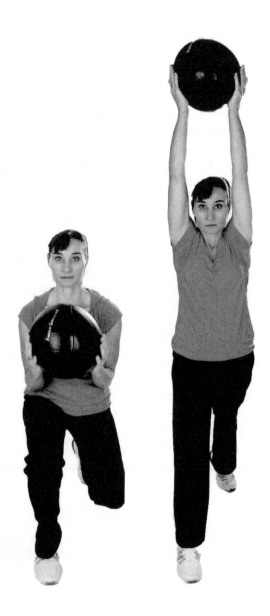

Chops

1. Use medicine ball appropriate for your fitness level. Choose the amount of weight based on your upper body strength.
2. Start standing with your feet shoulder width apart and your chest up.
3. Hold medicine ball securely in front of body.
4. Holding ball in front of body, perform a squat. Bend at your hips and knees as you squat
5. Push your hips back to bring your thighs to nearly parallel to the ground. Make sure your knees remain in line with your hips and toes. Do not allow your knees to move laterally, from side to side. Make sure your knees do not go forward beyond your toes.
6. As you rise from the squat bring the medicine ball forward and then up above your head.
7. Hold briefly in this position and then squat again while simultaneously moving your arms with the ball to the lower position in front of your body.

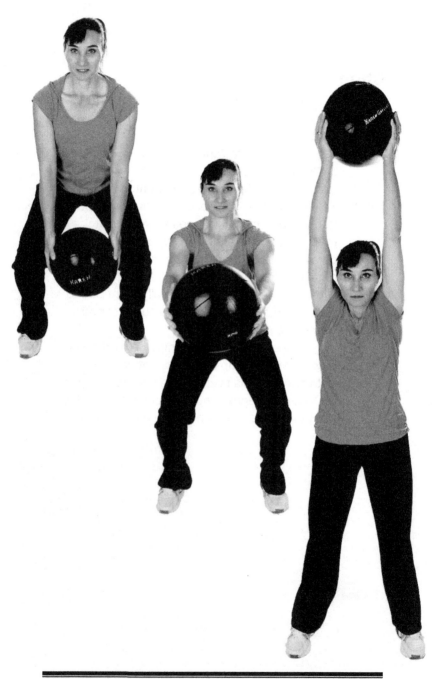

Circles

1. Use medicine ball appropriate for your fitness level. Choose the amount of weight based on your upper body strength.
2. Start standing with your feet shoulder width apart and your chest up.
3. Hold medicine ball securely in front of body.
4. Holding ball in front of body, perform a squat. Bend at your hips and knees as you squat
5. Push your hips back to bring your thighs to nearly parallel to the ground. Make sure your knees remain in line with your hips and toes. Do not allow your knees to move laterally, from side to side. Make sure your knees do not go forward beyond your toes.
6. As you rise from the squat bring the medicine ball to the right side and then up above your head.
7. Lower the medicine ball to the left side as you squat again.
8. Continue with a circular motion as you squat and rise.
9. Perform circles to the left for the same number of repetitions as you did to the right.

Legs Plus Workouts

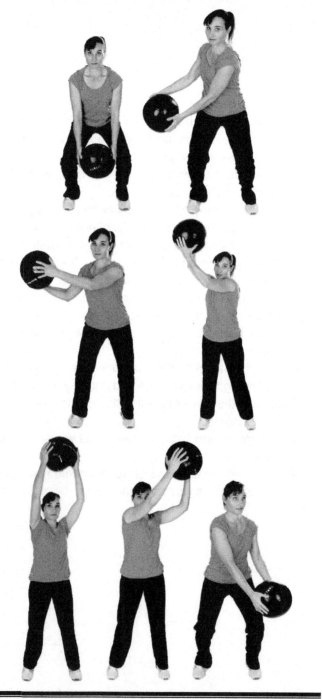

Figure 8 (Two circles.)

1. Use medicine ball appropriate for your fitness level. Choose the amount of weight based on your upper body strength.
2. Start standing with your feet shoulder width apart and your chest up.
3. Hold medicine ball securely in front of body.
4. Holding ball in front of body, perform a squat. Bend at your hips and knees as you squat
1. Push your hips back to bring your thighs to nearly parallel to the ground. Make sure your knees remain in line with your hips and toes. Do not allow your knees to move laterally, from side to side. Make sure your knees do not go forward beyond your toes.
2. As you rise from the squat bring the medicine ball to the right side and then up above your head.
3. Lower the medicine ball forward so that it is in front of your chest and immediately bring it to the left thigh.
4. Squat each time the ball is lowered. Rise each time the ball is lifted.
5. Once the ball touches the thigh lift it up towards the left, above your head, forward , and to the right thigh.
6. Continue the figure 8 pattern. It will feel like you are forming two circles side by side.

Legs Plus Workouts

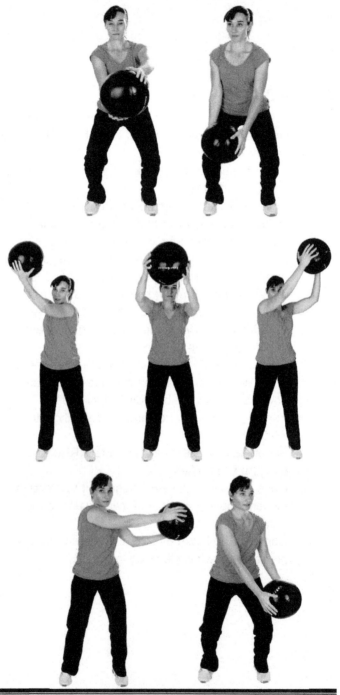

LEGS PLUS WORKOUT SEVEN

Legs Plus Workouts

Side Lunge with Front / Side Raise

1. Use dumbbells appropriate for your fitness level. Choose the amount of weight based on your upper body strength.
2. Start standing with your feet together and your chest up.
3. Hold weights securely at your thighs with palms facing body.
4. Take a large step with right foot out to the right side.
5. As right foot makes contact with the floor, bend the knee and at the hip to form a side lunge position.
6. As the leg is stepping to the side, bring left arm forward and up to the height of your shoulder. Bring your right arm up to the side and the height of your shoulder. Arms will be in an L position.
7. Keep your elbows relaxed, not locked.
8. Bottom position will be a side lunge, right leg bent at near 90 degrees with left leg straight. Your arms will be in an L position at shoulder height.
9. Hold briefly in this position.
10. Return to starting position by standing back up to bring your legs together and your hands back down to your thighs.
11. Repeat this exercise with the left leg stepping to the left side with the opposite arms rising to shoulder height.

Legs Plus Workouts

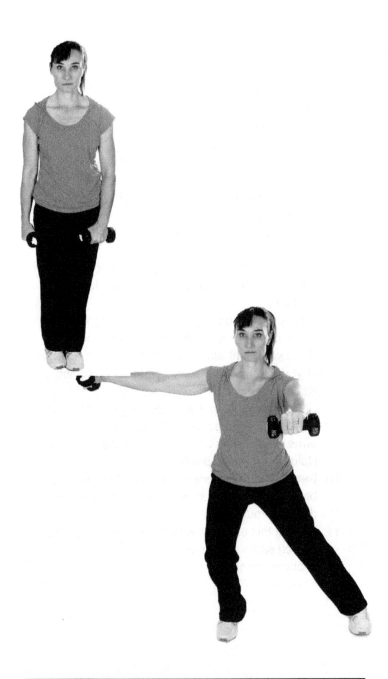

Squat and Press with Dumbbells

1. Use dumbbells appropriate for your fitness level. Choose the amount of weight based on your upper body strength.
2. Start standing with your feet shoulder width apart and your chest up.
3. Hold dumbbells securely in front of shoulders to start.
4. Bend at your hips and knees as you squat
5. Push your hips back to bring your thighs to nearly parallel to the ground. Make sure your knees remain in line with your hips and toes. Do not allow your knees to move laterally, from side to side. Make sure your knees do not go forward beyond your toes.
6. As you rise from the squat press the dumbbells up above your head.
7. Hold briefly in this position and then squat again while simultaneously moving your arms with the dumbbells to the lower position in front of your shoulders.
8. Repeat the rise and press the dumbbells up towards the ceiling.

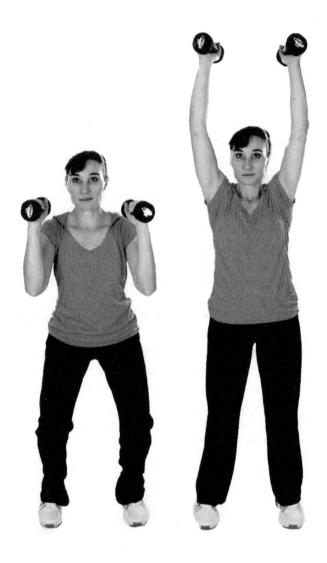

Lunge and Curl

1. Use dumbbells appropriate for your fitness level. Choose the amount of weight based on your upper body strength.
2. Start standing with your feet together and your chest up. Take a step forward with your right foot, as far as comfortable without losing balance.
3. Hold dumbbells securely at your sides.
4. Keeping your chest up, bend both knees so that your back knee drops close to the floor.
5. The goal is to bring the knee on your left leg close to floor behind you without actually touching the floor. Your left foot will remain on the floor.
6. The thigh on your right leg will be nearly parallel to the floor at the bottom of the exercise.
7. Bottom position will be a lunge, both legs bent at near 90 degrees with back knee close to floor. The dumbbells will be at your sides.
8. Hold briefly in this position.
9. Begin to rise back up and simultaneously curl the dumbbells so that your arms bend to a 90 degree angle. Keep your elbows pressed on your body so that you are performing a controlled biceps curl.
10. Stay tall, but do not lean back.
11. Repeat this exercise with the other leg in front.

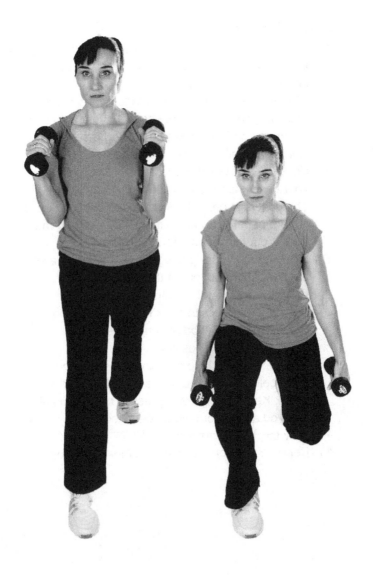

Legs Plus Workouts

Chops

1. Use medicine ball appropriate for your fitness level. Choose the amount of weight based on your upper body strength.
2. Start standing with your feet shoulder width apart and your chest up.
3. Hold medicine ball securely in front of body.
4. Holding ball in front of body, perform a squat. Bend at your hips and knees as you squat
5. Push your hips back to bring your thighs to nearly parallel to the ground. Make sure your knees remain in line with your hips and toes. Do not allow your knees to move laterally, from side to side. Make sure your knees do not go forward beyond your toes.
6. As you rise from the squat bring the medicine ball forward and then up above your head.
7. Hold briefly in this position and then squat again while simultaneously moving your arms with the ball to the lower position in front of your body.

Legs Plus Workouts

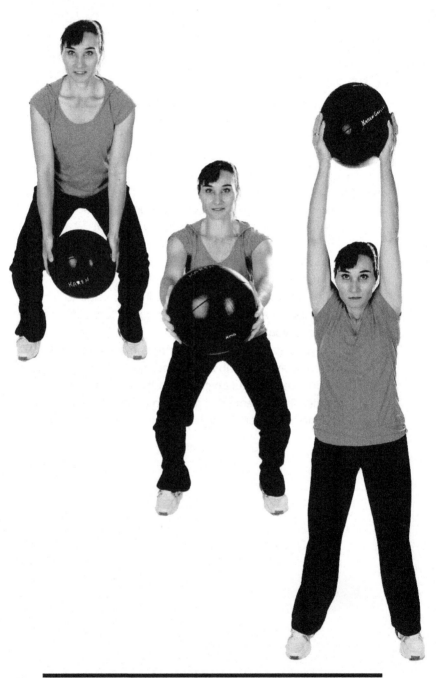

Lunge with Press with Dumbbells

1. Use dumbbells appropriate for your fitness level. Choose the amount of weight based on your upper body strength.
2. Start standing with your feet together and your chest up. Take a step forward with your right foot, as far as comfortable without losing balance.
3. Hold dumbbells securely at your shoulders.
4. Keeping your chest up, bend both knees so that your back knee drops close to the floor.
5. The goal is to bring the knee on your left leg close to floor behind you without actually touching the floor. Your left foot will remain on the floor.
6. The thigh on your right leg will be nearly parallel to the floor at the bottom of the exercise.
7. Bottom position will be a lunge, both legs bent at near 90 degrees with back knee close to floor. The dumbbells will be at your shoulders.
8. Hold briefly in this position.
9. Begin to rise back up and simultaneously press the dumbbells up towards the ceiling so that the dumbbells are high above your head. Do not lock your elbows at the top.
10. Stay tall, but do not lean back.
11. Repeat this exercise with the other leg in front.

Legs Plus Workouts

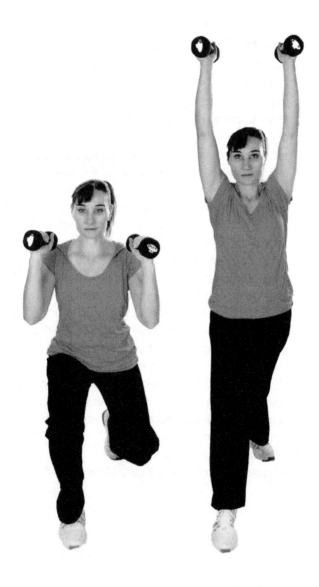

Legs Plus Workouts

Circles

1. Use medicine ball appropriate for your fitness level. Choose the amount of weight based on your upper body strength.
2. Start standing with your feet shoulder width apart and your chest up.
3. Hold medicine ball securely in front of body.
4. Holding ball in front of body, perform a squat. Bend at your hips and knees as you squat
5. Push your hips back to bring your thighs to nearly parallel to the ground. Make sure your knees remain in line with your hips and toes. Do not allow your knees to move laterally, from side to side. Make sure your knees do not go forward beyond your toes.
6. As you rise from the squat bring the medicine ball to the right side and then up above your head.
7. Lower the medicine ball to the left side as you squat again.
8. Continue with a circular motion as you squat and rise.
9. Perform circles to the left for the same number of repetitions as you did to the right.

Legs Plus Workouts

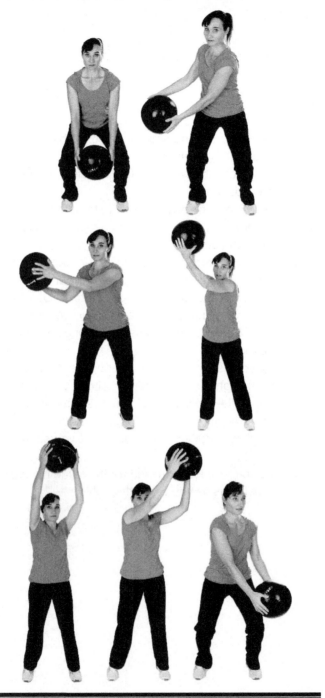

LEGS PLUS WORKOUT EIGHT

Legs Plus Workouts

Legs Plus Workouts

Chops

1. Use medicine ball appropriate for your fitness level. Choose the amount of weight based on your upper body strength.
2. Start standing with your feet shoulder width apart and your chest up.
3. Hold medicine ball securely in front of body.
4. Holding ball in front of body, perform a squat. Bend at your hips and knees as you squat
5. Push your hips back to bring your thighs to nearly parallel to the ground. Make sure your knees remain in line with your hips and toes. Do not allow your knees to move laterally, from side to side. Make sure your knees do not go forward beyond your toes.
6. As you rise from the squat bring the medicine ball forward and then up above your head.
7. Hold briefly in this position and then squat again while simultaneously moving your arms with the ball to the lower position in front of your body.

Legs Plus Workouts

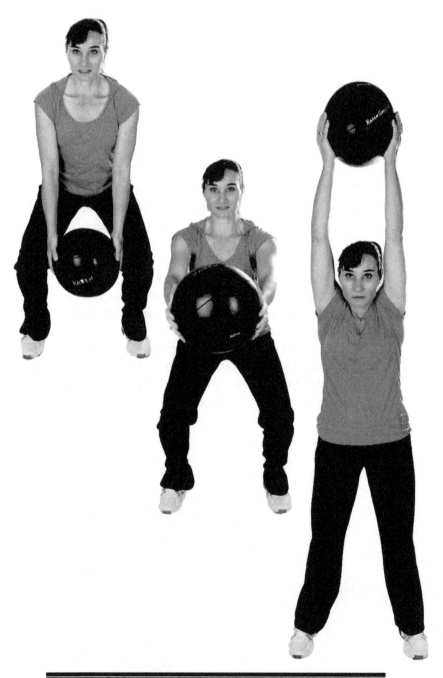

Circles

1. Use medicine ball appropriate for your fitness level. Choose the amount of weight based on your upper body strength.
2. Start standing with your feet shoulder width apart and your chest up.
3. Hold medicine ball securely in front of body.
4. Holding ball in front of body, perform a squat. Bend at your hips and knees as you squat
5. Push your hips back to bring your thighs to nearly parallel to the ground. Make sure your knees remain in line with your hips and toes. Do not allow your knees to move laterally, from side to side. Make sure your knees do not go forward beyond your toes.
6. As you rise from the squat bring the medicine ball to the right side and then up above your head.
7. Lower the medicine ball to the left side as you squat again.
8. Continue with a circular motion as you squat and rise.
9. Perform circles to the left for the same number of repetitions as you did to the right.

Legs Plus Workouts

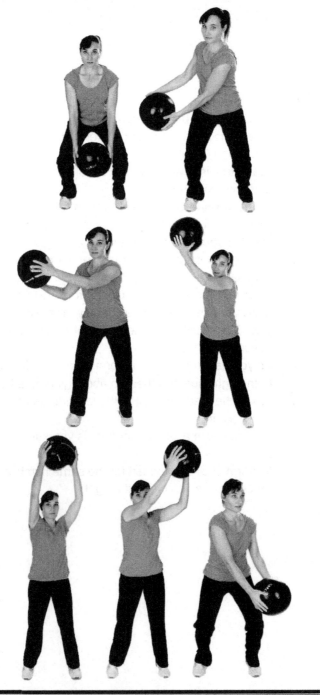

Figure 8 (Two circles.)

5. Use medicine ball appropriate for your fitness level. Choose the amount of weight based on your upper body strength.
6. Start standing with your feet shoulder width apart and your chest up.
7. Hold medicine ball securely in front of body.
8. Holding ball in front of body, perform a squat. Bend at your hips and knees as you squat
7. Push your hips back to bring your thighs to nearly parallel to the ground. Make sure your knees remain in line with your hips and toes. Do not allow your knees to move laterally, from side to side. Make sure your knees do not go forward beyond your toes.
8. As you rise from the squat bring the medicine ball to the right side and then up above your head.
9. Lower the medicine ball forward so that it is in front of your chest and immediately bring it to the left thigh.
10. Squat each time the ball is lowered. Rise each time the ball is lifted.
11. Once the ball touches the thigh lift it up towards the left, above your head, forward , and to the right thigh.
12. Continue the figure 8 pattern. It will feel like you are forming two circles side by side.

Legs Plus Workouts

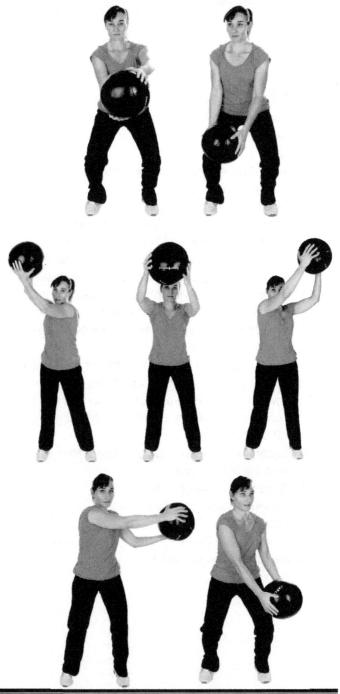

Driving

1. Use medicine ball appropriate for your fitness level. Choose the amount of weight based on your upper body strength.
2. Start standing with your feet shoulder width apart and your chest up.
3. Hold medicine ball securely in front of body at chest height.
4. Holding ball in front of body, perform a squat. Bend at your hips and knees as you squat
5. Push your hips back to bring your thighs to nearly parallel to the ground. Make sure your knees remain in line with your hips and toes. Do not allow your knees to move laterally, from side to side. Make sure your knees do not go forward beyond your toes.
6. Hold the squat position with the ball at chest height during this exercise.
7. Rotate the ball so that your right hand is on top and your left hand is on the bottom.
8. Rotate the ball again so that your left hand is on top and right hand is on bottom. Continue to rotate the ball in a driving motion as you keep it at chest height in front of your body.

Legs Plus Workouts

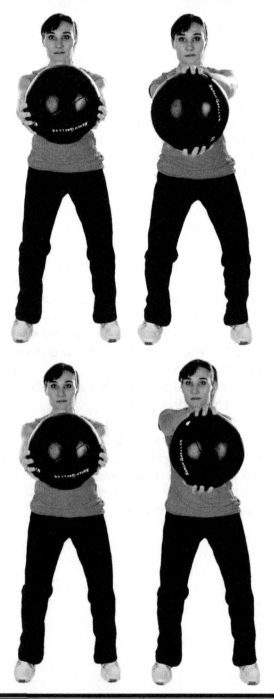

LEGS PLUS WORKOUT NINE

Squat with Iron Cross

1. Use dumbbells appropriate for your fitness level. Choose the amount of weight based on your upper body strength.
2. Start standing with your feet shoulder width apart and your chest up.
3. Hold weights securely at shoulder height with palms facing forward.
4. Bend at your hips and knees as you squat
5. Push your hips back to bring your thighs to nearly parallel to the ground. Make sure your knees remain in line with your hips and toes. Do not allow your knees to move laterally, from side to side. Make sure your knees do not go forward beyond your toes.
6. As you begin to squat, bring your hands towards each other in front of your chest.
7. Hold briefly in this position and then stand up while simultaneously moving your arms out to the sides and still at shoulder height.

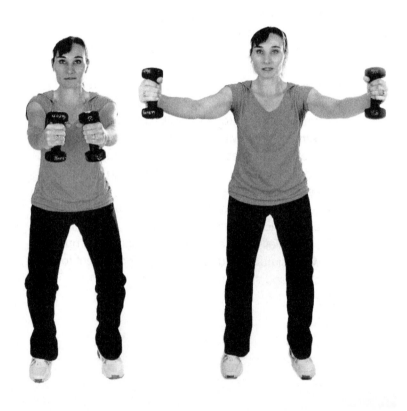

Legs Plus Workouts

Side Lunge with Front / Side Raise

1. Use dumbbells appropriate for your fitness level. Choose the amount of weight based on your upper body strength.
2. Start standing with your feet together and your chest up.
3. Hold weights securely at your thighs with palms facing body.
4. Take a large step with right foot out to the right side.
5. As right foot makes contact with the floor, bend the knee and at the hip to form a side lunge position.
6. As the leg is stepping to the side, bring left arm forward and up to the height of your shoulder. Bring your right arm up to the side and the height of your shoulder. Arms will be in an L position.
7. Keep your elbows relaxed, not locked.
8. Bottom position will be a side lunge, right leg bent at near 90 degrees with left leg straight. Your arms will be in an L position at shoulder height.
9. Hold briefly in this position.
10. Return to starting position by standing back up to bring your legs together and your hands back down to your thighs.
11. Repeat this exercise with the left leg stepping to the left side with the opposite arms rising to shoulder height.

Legs Plus Workouts

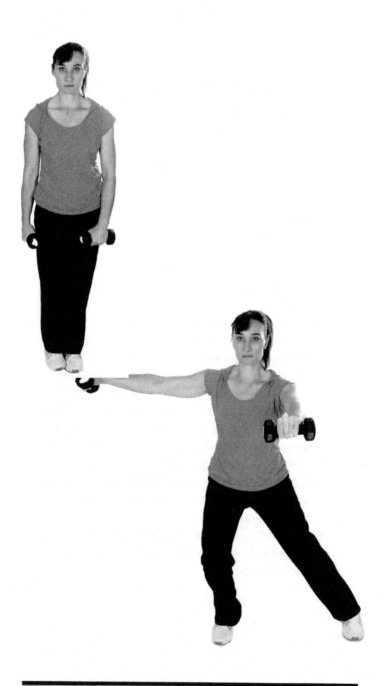

Legs Plus Workouts

Squat and Upright Row

1. Use dumbbell appropriate for your fitness level. Choose the amount of weight based on your upper body strength.
2. Start standing with your feet shoulder width apart and your chest up.
3. Hold dumbbell securely in front of your body to start. Hold the inner portion of the end, rounded part of the dumbbell.
4. Bend at your hips and knees as you squat
5. Push your hips back to bring your thighs to nearly parallel to the ground. Make sure your knees remain in line with your hips and toes. Do not allow your knees to move laterally, from side to side. Make sure your knees do not go forward beyond your toes.
6. As you rise from the squat pull the dumbbell up towards your ribs. Pull to a comfortable height, no higher than chest.
7. Hold briefly in this position and then squat again while simultaneously moving your arms with the dumbbell to the lower position.

Legs Plus Workouts

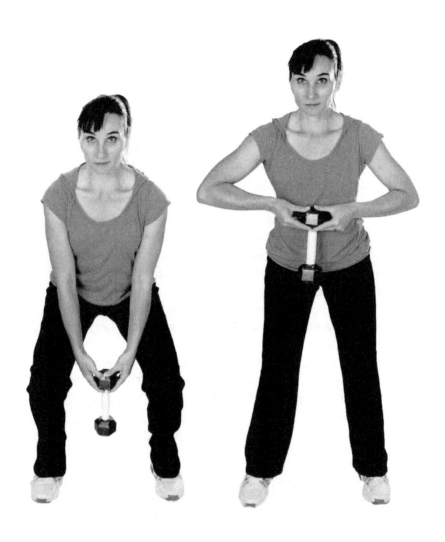

Lunge with Press with Dumbbells

1. Use dumbbells appropriate for your fitness level. Choose the amount of weight based on your upper body strength.
2. Start standing with your feet together and your chest up. Take a step forward with your right foot, as far as comfortable without losing balance.
3. Hold dumbbells securely at your shoulders.
4. Keeping your chest up, bend both knees so that your back knee drops close to the floor.
5. The goal is to bring the knee on your left leg close to floor behind you without actually touching the floor. Your left foot will remain on the floor.
6. The thigh on your right leg will be nearly parallel to the floor at the bottom of the exercise.
7. Bottom position will be a lunge, both legs bent at near 90 degrees with back knee close to floor. The dumbbells will be at your shoulders.
8. Hold briefly in this position.
9. Begin to rise back up and simultaneously press the dumbbells up towards the ceiling so that the dumbbells are high above your head. Do not lock your elbows at the top.
10. Stay tall, but do not lean back.
11. Repeat this exercise with the other leg in front.

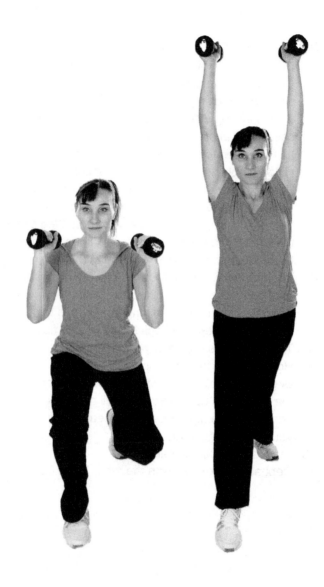

Chops

1. Use medicine ball appropriate for your fitness level. Choose the amount of weight based on your upper body strength.
2. Start standing with your feet shoulder width apart and your chest up.
3. Hold medicine ball securely in front of body.
4. Holding ball in front of body, perform a squat. Bend at your hips and knees as you squat
5. Push your hips back to bring your thighs to nearly parallel to the ground. Make sure your knees remain in line with your hips and toes. Do not allow your knees to move laterally, from side to side. Make sure your knees do not go forward beyond your toes.
6. As you rise from the squat bring the medicine ball forward and then up above your head.
7. Hold briefly in this position and then squat again while simultaneously moving your arms with the ball to the lower position in front of your body.

Legs Plus Workouts

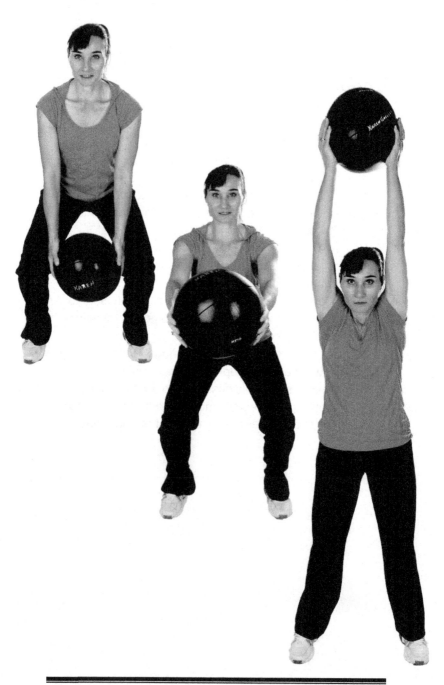

Mountain Climbers

1. Start in a push up position.
2. Your hands may be on the floor or on dumbbells that will not roll out.
3. Your body will be straight or slightly rounded, as long as your core does not fall towards the floor.
4. Bring your right knee in towards your chest, keeping your foot off the floor.
5. Switch your legs, returning the right leg to the starting position and then bringing the left knee in towards your chest.
6. You can think of this exercise as alternating knee ins or as a running motion if you are comfortable moving quickly.

Legs Plus Workouts

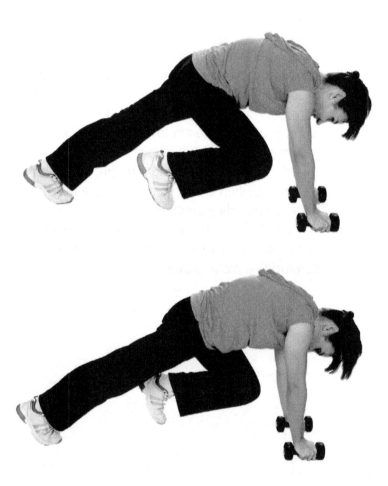

LEGS PLUS WORKOUT TEN

Legs Plus Workouts

Step Up with Knee Lift

1. Stand in front of step no higher than the height of your knee.
2. Place your right foot on the step to start.
3. Bend both arms to a 90 degree angle.
4. Lift the left arm forward and up so that you will be using the opposite arm to leg motion.
5. Step up onto the step and lift your left knee towards the ceiling, keeping the left leg bent.
6. S you step up you will switch arms as if performing a marching or running motion.
7. At the top of the exercise you will be on the step with your left leg up and right arm in front.
8. Bring the left foot back towards the floor and bend that knee as your foot makes contact with the floor.
9. Repeat the exercise with the left foot on the step for the same number of repetitions as you did on the right.

Legs Plus Workouts

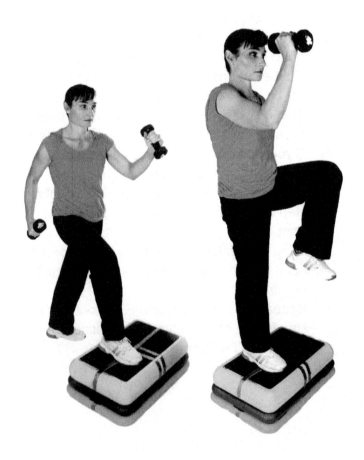

Lunge with Crossover

1. Use medicine ball appropriate for your fitness level. Choose the amount of weight based on your upper body strength.
2. Start standing with your feet together and your chest up. Take a step forward with your right foot, as far as comfortable without losing balance.
3. Hold medicine ball securely in front of your body, to start. Once you bend your legs, the medicine ball should be inside your front thigh.
4. Keeping your chest up, bend both knees so that your back knee drops close to the floor.
5. The goal is to bring the knee on your left leg close to floor behind you without actually touching the floor. Your left foot will remain on the floor.
6. The thigh on your right leg will be nearly parallel to the floor at the bottom of the exercise.
7. Bottom position will be a lunge, both legs bent at near 90 degrees with back knee close to floor. The medicine ball will be in front of your body, inside your front thigh.
8. Hold briefly in this position.
9. Begin to rise up and simultaneously lift the ball forward and then above your opposite shoulder.
10. Stay tall, but do not lean back.
11. Repeat this exercise with the other leg in front.

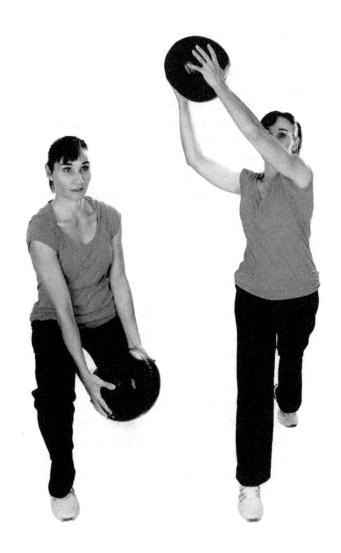

Reverse Lunge with Front / Side Raise

1. Use dumbbells appropriate for your fitness level. Choose the amount of weight based on your upper body strength.
2. Start standing with your feet together and your chest up.
3. Hold weights securely at your thighs with palms facing body.
4. Lift left foot from floor and reach back with that foot. The goal is to bring the knee on your left leg close to floor behind you without actually touching the floor. Your left foot will touch the floor.
5. Bend the right leg as your left knee gets close to the floor.
6. As the leg is going back, bring left arm forward and up to the height of your shoulder. Bring your right arm up to the side and the height of your shoulder. Arms will be in an L position.
7. Keep your elbows relaxed, not locked.
8. Bottom position will be a lunge, both legs bent at near 90 degrees with back knee close to floor. Your arms will be in an L position at shoulder height.
9. Hold briefly in this position.
10. Return to starting position by standing back up to bring your legs together and your hands back down to your thighs.
11. Repeat this exercise with the right leg stepping back and the opposite arms.

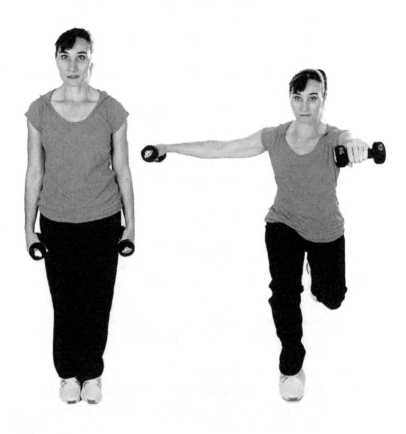

Legs Plus Workouts

Lunge and Press

1. Use medicine ball appropriate for your fitness level. Choose the amount of weight based on your upper body strength.
2. Start standing with your feet together and your chest up. Take a step forward with your right foot, as far as comfortable without losing balance.
3. Hold medicine ball securely in front of your chest.
4. Keeping your chest up, bend both knees so that your back knee drops close to the floor.
5. The goal is to bring the knee on your left leg close to floor behind you without actually touching the floor. Your left foot will remain on the floor.
6. The thigh on your right leg will be nearly parallel to the floor at the bottom of the exercise.
7. Bottom position will be a lunge, both legs bent at near 90 degrees with back knee close to floor. The medicine ball will be in front of your chest.
8. Hold briefly in this position.
9. Begin to rise back up and simultaneously lift the ball above your head.
10. Stay tall, but do not lean back.
11. Repeat this exercise with the other leg in front.

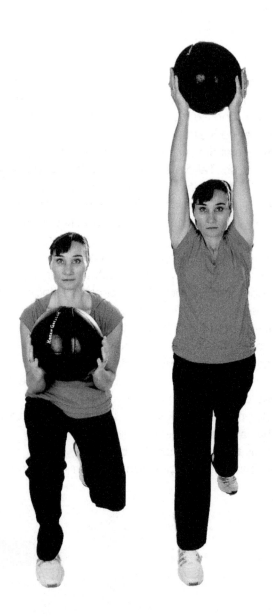

Side Lunge with Front / Side Raise

1. Use dumbbells appropriate for your fitness level. Choose the amount of weight based on your upper body strength.
2. Start standing with your feet together and your chest up.
3. Hold weights securely at your thighs with palms facing body.
4. Take a large step with right foot out to the right side.
5. As right foot makes contact with the floor, bend the knee and at the hip to form a side lunge position.
6. As the leg is stepping to the side, bring left arm forward and up to the height of your shoulder. Bring your right arm up to the side and the height of your shoulder. Arms will be in an L position.
7. Keep your elbows relaxed, not locked.
8. Bottom position will be a side lunge, right leg bent at near 90 degrees with left leg straight. Your arms will be in an L position at shoulder height.
9. Hold briefly in this position.
10. Return to starting position by standing back up to bring your legs together and your hands back down to your thighs.
11. Repeat this exercise with the left leg stepping to the left side with the opposite arms rising to shoulder height.

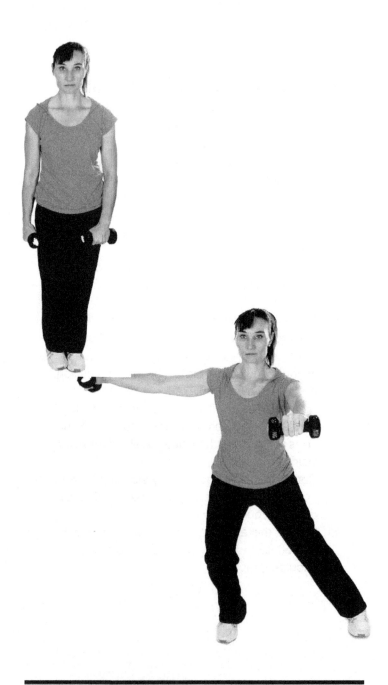

About the Author

Karen Goeller has educated thousands in the fitness and gymnastics industries with her books, articles, and in person. She has been training athletes since 1978 and adults since 1985. Karen Goeller is the author of more gymnastics books than anyone in the USA.

Karen started writing books after she was involved in an accident in 2000 and suffered permanent spinal damage. She stopped coaching gymnastics and left her advertising job. To remain involved in gymnastics and fitness, Karen turned to writing. "I felt like I had a ton of information in my head that was not being used. I knew it was the perfect time to pass on this knowledge and writing books was the perfect avenue."

Karen Goeller's first book, "Over 75 Drills and Conditioning Exercises" was used to create countless successful fitness and gymnastics training programs. Her books have been called the "most useful on the market."

Karen's most recent books are the Swing Set Fitness books. They were completed with Brian Dowd, Karen's nephew, who is a physical education teacher. It wasn't until the Swing Set Fitness books that Karen started to make good progress with her

Legs Plus Workouts

physical rehabilitation. Karen shared, "I finally feel like myself again. I knew I was getting stronger, mentally and physically." When asked if she is healed from the accident, Karen replied, "I am still injured, but that no longer defines me."

Karen has produced NY State Champions, National TOPS Team Athletes, and Empire State Games Athletes. Three National Champions are from Karen's gymnastics club. This success was after her 1991 cancer surgery. The cancer surgery was a success, but Karen was left with **lymphedema** in her leg. She was forced to keep her leg elevated or in motion 24/7 and in a compression stocking.

Karen Goeller and her athletes have been featured in the media since the 1990's. He has appeared on Good Morning America, GoodDay NY, Eyewitness News, and NY Views (old show) among others. They have also been featured in The NY Times, NY Newsday, Brooklyn Bridge Magazine, and Interview Magazine, and most of the Brooklyn, NY neighborhood newspapers. More recently Karen has been featured on Erin Ley Radio, Lynn Johnson Radio, I Run MY Body Radio, Late Night with Johnny Potenza TV, Talkin' Health with Joe Kasper Radio, the Coast Star, Asbury Park Press, Observer/Reporter, Staten Island Advance, and Inside Gymnastics Magazine. Karen has worked for world famous Olympic coach, Bela Karolyi and was his first female camp director.

Before earning her BA Degree, Karen's education included training as an EMT, Physical Therapist, and Nutritionist. She has had certifications such as EMT-

Legs Plus Workouts

D, Nutritional Analysis, Fitness Trainer, many USAG certifications, and the NSCA-CSCS certification.

For more training programs visit **www.Legs-Plus.com** and **www.SwingSetFitness.com**. You can get general fitness, speed & agility, gymnastics conditioning, golf conditioning, and other exercise programs as well as articles.

For more information on the author, Karen Goeller, CSCS visit **www.KarenGoeller.com**.

For more information on the photographer, visit **www.BossioPhotography.com**.

Books by Karen Goeller

1. Legs Plus Workouts
2. Gymnastics Lessons Learned: Life Lessons through Gymnastics
3. Lymphedema: Sentenced to Life in Bed, but I Escaped
4. Fitness on a Swing Set
5. Fitness on a Swing Set with Training Programs
6. Swing Set Workouts
7. One Swing Set Workout
8. Gymnastics Drills and Conditioning Exercises
9. Handstand Drills and Conditioning Exercises
10. Gymnastics Drills: Walkover, Limber, Back Handspring
11. Gymnastics Conditioning for the Legs and Ankles
12. Gymnastics Journal: My Scores, My Goals, My Dreams
13. Most Frequently Asked Questions about Gymnastics
14. Fitness Journal: My Goals, Training, and Success
15. Strength Training Journal
16. Gymnastics Conditioning: Five Conditioning Workouts
17. Gymnastics Conditioning: Tumbling Conditioning

Karen has also written countless articles and exercise programs.

www.GymnasticsBooks.com
www.KarenGoeller.com

Legs Plus Workouts

Made in the USA
Middletown, DE
12 March 2023

26628258R00086